MW00960910

Disclaimer

This book is intended to help people become better informed medical consumers. The information in this book is intended to supplement, not replace, the medical advice of a trained health care professional. No mention or description of uses of drugs listed herein should be construed as an endorsement of those uses or drugs. Only a physician can prescribe drugs and their precise dosages. All matters regarding your health require medical supervision. The authors and publisher disclaim any liability arising directly or indirectly from use of this book.

Notice of rights

The information in this book is distributed on an "As Is" basis without warranty. While every precaution has been taken in the preparation of he book, neither the author nor the publisher shall have any liability to any person or entity with respect to any loss or damage caused or alleged to be caused directly or indirectly by the instructions contained in this book or by the products described in it.

Trademarks

Many of the designations used by manufacturers and sellers to distinguish their products are claimed as trademarks. Where those designations appear in this book, and the publisher was aware of a trademark claim, the designations appear as requested by the owner of the trademark. All other product names and services identified throughout this book are used in editorial fashion only and for the benefit of such companies with no intention of infringement of the trademark. No such use, or the use of any trade name, is intended to convey endorsement or other affiliation with this book.

Table of Contents

Your feedback is invaluable to us

If you recently bought this book, we would love to hear from you! You can do this by writing a review on amazon (or the online store where you purchased this book) about your last purchase! As part of our continual service improvement process, we love to hear real client experiences and feedback.

How does it work?
To post a review on Amazon, just log in to your account and click on the Create Your Own Review button (under Customer Reviews) of the relevant product page. You can find examples of product reviews in Amazon. If you purchased from another online store, simply follow their procedures.

Why use this book?

Everyone should ask questions when getting a prescription. This is especially important when your doctor or other health care professional prescribes you Clobetasol Propionate.

What should you ask?

Your health depends on good communication, but which questions to ask your doctor? Having the right questions is the answer.

Asking questions and providing information to your doctor and other care providers can improve your care. Talking with your doctor builds trust and leads to better satisfaction, quality, safety and results.

Asking questions is key to good communication with your doctor. If you do not ask questions, he or she may assume you already know the answer or that you do not want more information. Do not wait for the doctor to raise a specific question or subject; he or she may not know it is important to you. Be proactive. Ask questions.

Effective health care is a team effort. You are part of this team and play an important role. One of the best ways to communicate with your doctor and health care team is by asking questions. Since time is limited when you have your medical appointments, you will feel less rushed when you prepare your questions before your appointment.

Your doctor wants your questions. Doctors know a lot about a lot of things, but they do not always know everything about you, what you want to know or what is best for you.

Your questions give your doctor and health care professionals important information about you, like your most important health care concerns.

That is why they need you to speak up.

How to use this book?

When you meet with your doctor or other members of your health care team, you will hear a lot of information. It helps to think ahead of time of the things you want to know and to highlight the questions in this book you want to ask and take this book with you to your appointments.

This book contains questions you may want to ask your doctor. You should use the questions that fit your situation, and skip those that do not apply.

This book offers many ways that you can ask questions and get your health care needs met. With this book you will have numerous simple questions that can help you take better care of yourself, feel better, and get the right care at the right time.

Doctors and medical professionals want to know your questions to help them take better care of you and offer advice to get your most pressing questions answered.

Be prepared for your next medical appointment. Take this book with you if you are getting a checkup, want to discuss a problem or health condition, are getting a prescription, or talk about a medical test or surgery and be sure to write down the answers your health care professional provides for you in this book.

Whatever the reason for your appointment, it is important to be prepared.

Take charge of your health. Ask your health care providers questions and learn about the Clobetasol Propionate medicine you take.

BEGINNING OF THE QUESTION CHAPTERS:

CHAPTER #1: WHO:

1. Who makes this Clobetasol Propionate medication?

Notes:

2. Who is eligible to receive Clobetasol Propionate prescription drug help?

Notes:

3. Can I use this app I found?

Notes:

4. Do I need this particular Clobetasol Propionate medication?

Notes:

5. Will Clobetasol Propionate medication be the proper strength?

Notes:

6. Should I buy generic Clobetasol Propionate prescription medications?

Notes:

7. Can Clobetasol Propionate prescription drugs cause problems during pregnancy?

Notes:

8. What if I am out of the country and lose my Clobetasol Propionate prescription medications?

Notes:

9. How can a wholesome mud-bath help my condition, and what is the effect on my Clobetasol Propionate prescription drugs?

Notes:

10. How will the treatment effect the medications that I currently take for _____?

Notes:

11. Are there any risks or side effects?

Notes:

12. When in care who is responsible for the MAR (Medication Administration Records), who can put information on to it and make changes?

Notes:

13. Who is validating my Clobetasol Propionate prescription drugs to make sure I am taking the correct pills?

Notes:

14. Are there any risks involved in having this test?

Notes:

15. Who gets to see the Clobetasol Propionate prescription drug information submitted in my patient medical questionnaire?

Notes:

16. Who is qualified to receive Clobetasol Propionate prescription drug help?

Notes:

17. So who approves these Clobetasol Propionate medications?

Notes:

18. Are there any side effects associated with this Clobetasol Propionate medication that I should know about?

Notes:

19. Who typically uses Clobetasol Propionate prescription drugs, and where do they get them?

Notes:

20. Can you slow down and keep it simple?

Notes:

21. Is this worth getting Clobetasol Propionate medication for?

Notes:

22. Do I have to pay for my own Clobetasol Propionate prescription drugs?

Notes:

23. Is it possible to start with a solution which is natural and effective and less expensive than Clobetasol Propionate prescription medication?

Notes:

24. What happens if I am willing to try new medications if the current Clobetasol Propionate ones are not working?

Notes:

25. Would I need Clobetasol Propionate prescription drugs that are not covered by insurance?

Notes:

26. What is the safest prescription drug disposal method?

Notes:

27. If I am unable to comply with the treatment regimen, who else can administer Clobetasol Propionate medication?

Notes:

28. Who gets Clobetasol Propionate, and when?

Notes:

29. Are medication reminders only for prescription medications?

Notes:

30. I feel like I need more medication, will you as my doctor be able to support me with my requests?

Notes:

31. Who can get Medicare Clobetasol Propionate prescription drug coverage?

Notes:

32. Who is most susceptible to Clobetasol Propionate prescription drug abuse?

Notes:

33. They say _____ not to take this with Clobetasol Propionate prescription medication, but do you think it will hurt me?

Notes:

34. What exactly is this Clobetasol Propionate medication for in my case and how do you think it is working so well?

Notes:

35. Who is at risk for Clobetasol Propionate prescription drug addiction?

Notes:

36. Is there an Over-The-Counter Medication that helps or maybe even can replace my Clobetasol Propionate Prescription Medication?

Notes:

37. Who can assist with Clobetasol Propionate medication reminders?

Notes:

38. Who should NOT take Clobetasol Propionate medication?

Notes:

39. What prescription drugs do I need covered?

Notes:

40. Is the answer in natural supplements, in Clobetasol Propionate prescription medications or some combination of both?

Notes:

41. Has anyone ever used this Clobetasol Propionate medication?

Notes:

42. Can all doctors prescribe Clobetasol Propionate Prescription Medication?

Notes:

43. How do you help someone who has a Clobetasol Propionate prescription drugs addiction?

Notes:

44. Who is accountable for my Clobetasol Propionate prescription drug use?

Notes:

45. Are there any other medicines that can help me but without any side effects?

Notes:

46. Do I need to take Clobetasol Propionate medications?

Notes:

47. What is the effect of my Clobetasol Propionate use if I smoke?

Notes:

48. Who can I contact if I want to meet with a specialist for long-term Clobetasol Propionate medication management on an ongoing basis?

Notes:

49. Who can join a Medicare Clobetasol Propionate prescription drug plan?

Notes:

50. Has there been any follow up of those who have stopped taking Clobetasol Propionate medication?

Notes:

51. How do you prevent re-admission in case I forget to take my Clobetasol Propionate prescription medications. How do you help those who have problems following suggestions regarding eating habits, smoking, drinking, and taking drugs..?

Notes:

52. I'm taking prescription medication abroad, will this be covered if it is lost or I run out?

Notes:

53. Should I have a current emergency contact form and a list of health conditions and medications readily available?

Notes:

54. Are Clobetasol Propionate medications safe for young kids?

Notes:

55. What should you do if I've messed up with my Clobetasol Propionate medication?

Notes:

56. What is the Prescription Drug Monitoring Database and who is using it?

Notes:

57. Are there any drug interactions if Clobetasol Propionate is taken in combination with other medications?

Notes:

58. Are there other remedies, is there any relief other than Clobetasol Propionate Medication?

Notes:

59. Will I need any Clobetasol Propionate medication after surgery?

Notes:

CHAPTER #2: WHAT:

INTENT: What do I need to know about Clobetasol Propionate (What will it do for me and what can I expect.)

1. What are good reasons to not take my Clobetasol Propionate prescription medication?

Notes:

2. What exactly leads one to get dependent on Clobetasol Propionate prescription drugs?

Notes:

3. What if I am taking vitamins or over-the-counter drugs that could affect my Clobetasol Propionate prescription drugs?

Notes:

4. How will I benefit from working out in relation to my use of Clobetasol Propionate prescription medication, and what type of exercise would you recommend?

Notes:

5. What will be the net effect of Clobetasol Propionate medications for me?

Notes:

6. What lifestyle changes can change my condition?

Notes:

7. What medications are available to treat my condition?

Notes:

8. What happens if I stop using Clobetasol Propionate cold-turkey?

Notes:

9. What should I do if I miss my regular dose of Clobetasol Propionate?

Notes:

10. What about taking a new Clobetasol Propionate medication?

Notes:

11. What is Clobetasol Propionate prescription drug detox?

Notes:

12. What is the test for?

Notes:

13. What is Clobetasol Propionate medication for?

Notes:

14. What should I expect after a procedure in terms of soreness, what to watch for, Clobetasol Propionate medication, bathing, and level of activity?

Notes:

15. What Clobetasol Propionate medications are used?

Notes:

16. What is the evidence for this treatment?

Notes:

17. How do I book in to have the test and what is the usual waiting period?

Notes:

18. What are my Clobetasol Propionate medication options?

Notes:

19. What does this sign on my Clobetasol Propionate

prescription drug imply?

Notes:

20. What is my outcome?

Notes:

21. What are the signs and symptoms related to Clobetasol Propionate addiction?

Notes:

22. What side effects can Clobetasol Propionate medication cause?

Notes:

23. What about alcohol and its effect on Clobetasol Propionate prescription drugs?

Notes:

24. What do I need to know about making the most of this Clobetasol Propionate prescription?

Notes:

25. What will my Clobetasol Propionate medication do for me?

Notes:

26. What Clobetasol Propionate prescription drugs have serious side effects?

Notes:

27. What is the proper course of treatment for me?

Notes:

28. How do scientists determine whether the chemical compounds in Clobetasol Propionate prescription medications do what they're claimed to do?

Notes:

29. Will I need medication and what will it be, Clobetasol Propionate and/or anything else?

Notes:

30. What's the difference between all of the Clobetasol Propionate's class medications?

Notes:

31. What to eat, or what to use as a medication together with Clobetasol Propionate?

Notes:

32. What prescription drugs are you yourself taking?

Notes:

33. What if I have been taking Clobetasol Propionate medication with little to no relief?

Notes:

34. What are my options in relation to Clobetasol Propionate medication, surgical procedures or remedy?

Notes:

35. What will a negative result mean?

Notes:

36. What should I do if I experience side effects from the Clobetasol Propionate?

Notes:

37. What is the branded prescription drug fee?

Notes:

38. For what reasons would I have to be off Clobetasol Propionate medication and for how long?

Notes:

39. What's your go-to question for your own doctor?

Notes:

40. What's to lose by trying another Clobetasol Propionate class medication?

Notes:

41. What are the different treatment options?

Notes:

42. What are the important warnings for males taking Clobetasol Propionate?

Notes:

43. What other prescription drugs should I avoid while taking my Clobetasol Propionate medicines?

Notes:

44. Is treatment required, if so - what is it?

Notes:

45. What should I do if I have other prescription drug coverage and want to join Medicare First?

Notes:

46. What are some of the best non prescription medications I can give a try?

Notes:

47. What would you do if you were me?

Notes:

48. Is Clobetasol Propionate safe when breastfeeding, what are the effects on nursing?

Notes:

49. What can I expect from Clobetasol Propionate medication?

Notes:

50. What if I have an allergic reaction to Clobetasol Propionate?

Notes:

51. What about my regular medications, any interference with Clobetasol Propionate?

Notes:

52. What kind of resources do I have available to me?

Notes:

53. What kind of medication will I have to take, Clobetasol Propionate or anything else?

Notes:

54. What about my current medications or allergies and the effect on it of Clobetasol Propionate?

Notes:

55. What Clobetasol Propionate's class medication can I take best?

Notes:

56. What if my prescription Clobetasol Propionate medication is lost or stolen?

Notes:

57. Can you help me understand how much of my Clobetasol Propionate prescription drugs, equipment and services will be covered by my insurance and what I will have to pay?

Notes:

58. What if I have tried various home remedies, over-the-counter medications or even Clobetasol Propionate prescription medications with no help?

Notes:

59. What medications on the market, OTC or Clobetasol Propionate prescription, can become harmful over time and would be dangerous if used well past the expiration date?

Notes:

60. What medications have you yourself used in the past to make yourself better?

Notes:

61. What will a positive result mean?

Notes:

62. What happens if I don't do anything?

Notes:

63. What's the probability that my Clobetasol Propionate medication is causing my symptoms?

Notes:

64. What do you recommend to do with Clobetasol Propionate medication adherence being difficult for me since my busy life pulls me in multiple directions - can you help me understand the ramifications of non-adherence?

Notes:

65. What happens if I have to cut my Clobetasol Propionate pills in half to make them last longer or

skip a day of medication because I can't afford to buy it as often as it's prescribed?

Notes:

66. What is the safest way to dispose of unwanted medications?

Notes:

67. What can I do to prevent my condition from recurring or worsening?

Notes:

68. What Clobetasol Propionate-like medications are safe to take during pregnancy?

Notes:

69. What non-Clobetasol Propionate medications or vitamins should I take to speed up my healing?

Notes:

70. What is my Clobetasol Propionate prescription

drug benefit?

Notes:

71. What are the benefits of having the test?

Notes:

72. What is the effect of Clobetasol Propionate on infertility?

Notes:

73. What is the way to get my life back on track, without the unwanted side effects of Clobetasol Propionate prescription drugs?

Notes:

74. What about side effects of Clobetasol Propionate?

Notes:

75. What if I take Clobetasol Propionate prescription drugs and get little or no relief?

Notes:

76. What is a generic Clobetasol Propionate medication or drug, what does that term mean and what can it do for me?

Notes:

77. What would happen if I don't take the Clobetasol Propionate, would my health get worse?

Notes:

78. What could be a natural alternative to more over-the-counter and Clobetasol Propionate prescription drugs?

Notes:

79. What if Clobetasol Propionate medication has changed since the application form was sent in?

Notes:

80. What kind of expectations should I have?

Notes:

81. What really works as well as these Clobetasol Propionate medications, are there alternatives?

Notes:

82. What medications can Clobetasol Propionate interact with?

Notes:

83. What other drugs could interact with Clobetasol Propionate medication?

Notes:

84. What is a generic Clobetasol Propionate medication?

Notes:

85. What if I am unhappy with the results of Clobetasol Propionate medication?

Notes:

86. What about Clobetasol Propionate's interactions with my medications?

Notes:

87. Apart from Clobetasol Propionate medication, what are other components of your management plan?

Notes:

88. What is a 25/50 percent Clobetasol Propionate prescription drug plan?

Notes:

89. What are your experiences with Clobetasol Propionate prescription drugs?

Notes:

90. What is the best approach if I forget to take this Clobetasol Propionate medication?

Notes:

91. What is the easiest way to obtain the latest information about Clobetasol Propionate prescription drugs?

Notes:

92. What if the Clobetasol Propionate medications produce unwelcome or harmful effects?

Notes:

93. What is the effect of Clobetasol Propionate on drowsiness?

Notes:

94. What can I do to help win the war on prescription drug abuse?

Notes:

95. What are my options if I have difficulty paying for Clobetasol Propionate prescription drugs?

Notes:

96. What are my risks of accidentally taking an overdose of Clobetasol Propionate prescription drugs?

Notes:

97. What other Clobetasol Propionate-like medications are in this class?

Notes:

98. What else could I be doing to stay healthy and prevent disease?

Notes:

99. What happens with my prescriptions for Clobetasol Propionate medications while I am travelling overseas, how to get and fulfil those?

Notes:

100. What causes my condition?

Notes:

101. What are the Clobetasol Propionate medication side-effects?

Notes:

102. Is it possible that my employer may look at what Clobetasol Propionate prescription medications I'm taking?

Notes:

103. Besides Clobetasol Propionate medication, what else to do?

Notes:

104. What will happen if I don't have the treatment?

Notes:

105. What should I know about Clobetasol Propionate medication?

Notes:

106. What is the safest way to dispose of unused prescription Clobetasol Propionate medication?

Notes:

107. What does a Clobetasol Propionate medication error involve?

Notes:

108. What is a prescription drug error and how often and why do these errors occur??

Notes:

109. What sort of Clobetasol Propionate prescription drug benefit is included?

Notes:

110. What medications should I ask for?

Notes:

111. What are the adverse health effects from Clobetasol Propionate prescription drugs?

Notes:

112. What is are food or drinks you recommend not to be taken with Clobetasol Propionate prescription medications?

Notes:

113. Do I need to change what I eat or stop any Clobetasol Propionate medications before doing a test?

Notes:

114. What is the name of my Clobetasol Propionate medication?

Notes:

115. At what point would you recommend Clobetasol Propionate prescription drugs, alternative therapies, or surgery?

Notes:

116. What's next?

Notes:

117. How will you know what medications I am on?

Notes:

118. What sources can I trust?

Notes:

119. What is the name of my condition, are there any other names it's known by?

Notes:

120. What kind of Clobetasol Propionate medications do the varying plans offer and how much can I save?

Notes:

121. What types of Clobetasol Propionate medications

are available?

Notes:

122. What replacement medications can you suggest for Clobetasol Propionate?

Notes:

123. What types of vitamins and supplements should I be taking?

Notes:

124. What are other treatment options?

Notes:

125. What else can I do to treat my condition?

Notes:

126. What are the important warnings for females taking Clobetasol Propionate?

Notes:

127. What Clobetasol Propionate medication should I take?

Notes:

128. What is the nature of the Clobetasol Propionate medications prescribed?

Notes:

129. What can I do to remember to take my Clobetasol Propionate medication?

Notes:

130. What is the brand name for the drug Clobetasol Propionate?

Notes:

131. What are the side effects?

Notes:

132. What prescription medications or off the shelf medicinal products would cause ringing in the ears?

Notes:

133. What questions haven't I asked that I should have?

Notes:

134. What if Clobetasol Propionate medication makes me gain weight?

Notes:

135. What does my Clobetasol Propionate medication look like?

Notes:

136. In what way can mindfulness or meditation be useful?

Notes:

137. What sexual response side effects can I expect from these Clobetasol Propionate medications?

Notes:

138. What if I am currently taking some other prescription medications?

Notes:

139. What about Clobetasol Propionate prescription drug coverage?

Notes:

140. What can parents and other adults do to help prevent prescription drug abuse among youth?

Notes:

141. What if I'm already on medication and have side-effects from the Clobetasol Propionate?

Notes:

142. What are the causes of Clobetasol Propionate prescription drug abuse?

Notes:

143. What are the Clobetasol Propionate medications I can take?

Notes:

144. What if I'm taking other medication?

Notes:

145. What will this test tell us?

Notes:

146. I want to read more about my condition. What online sources should I trust?

Notes:

147. What are your thoughts on hypnotherapy and Clobetasol Propionate?

Notes:

148. What kind of experience with these issues do you have?

Notes:

149. What is the prescription drug of choice for breakthrough pain meds?

Notes:

150. In what situation would I need to go for counseling if I'm receiving medication treatment?

Notes:

151. What are the side effects of the Clobetasol Propionate medication?

Notes:

152. What's the best mix for me of home remedies, over the counter (OTC) drugs and ointments and Clobetasol Propionate prescription drugs?

Notes:

153. What should you, as my doctor, know before prescribing Clobetasol Propionate medication?

Notes:

154. What outcome should I expect?

Notes:

155. What are the dosages of the Clobetasol Propionate medication?

Notes:

156. What other sources are available, who can I talk to about this?

Notes:

157. What will happen to me without Clobetasol Propionate prescription drugs, diet, exercise, or nutritional supplements?

Notes:

CHAPTER #3: WHERE:

INTENT: Where to next (Where can I find more information. Do i need a second opionion. What happens with tests.)

1. Do I really need to take this Clobetasol Propionate medication?

Notes:

2. Can I drink alcohol while I am taking Clobetasol Propionate?

Notes:

3. What if I am currently without prescription drug coverage?

Notes:

4. Where can I get my Clobetasol Propionate prescription medications filled?

Notes:

5. Precisely what are some good reasons Clobetasol Propionate prescription drugs can be recommended?

Notes:

6. Where do I go if I've run out of money and desperately need Clobetasol Propionate medication or a medical procedure?

Notes:

7. Are there any side effects from taking nutritional supplements and Clobetasol Propionate prescription medications at the same time?

Notes:

8. Should I really use this Clobetasol Propionate medication?

Notes:

9. How do I use my insurance to get discounts on my Clobetasol Propionate prescription medication?

Notes:

10. Will you try and reach the primary reason for my problem before prescribing Clobetasol Propionate medications to solve my particular signs and symptoms?

Notes:

11. Could you write it down?

Notes:

12. Are there simpler - safer options?

Notes:

13. So, are Clobetasol Propionate prescription drugs safe?

Notes:

14. Is it likely to get worse, or is it likely to get better?

Notes:

15. Where can I find info about taking more than one prescription medications together with Clobetasol Propionate?

Notes:

16. Do you have Clobetasol Propionate prescription drugs I can take throughout the day?

Notes:

17. If remedies help, what is the nature of Clobetasol Propionate medications and where could one go to explore them?

Notes:

18. Is there anything I should do to help prevent my health issue?

Notes:

19. Can my Clobetasol Propionate medication be delivered if I don't attend appointments?

Notes:

20. If I am taking Clobetasol Propionate prescription medications can I take natural remedies?

Notes:

21. Can I travel to _____ with prescription drugs used as medication for my condition?

Notes:

22. Do I need to see any other health professionals - such as specialists - physiotherapists - dieticians or dentists?

Notes:

23. Will any supplements interact with my Clobetasol Propionate prescription drugs?

Notes:

24. Is there anything I can do to improve it myself?

Notes:

25. Are any medications I am taking likely to cause breast problems?

Notes:

26. Will Clobetasol Propionate medication control my symptoms adequately?

Notes:

27. Would increasing the dose of Clobetasol Propionate have a positive effect or would I be better off asking you to try some new medications?

Notes:

28. Which Clobetasol Propionate medications are addictive?

Notes:

29. Can I share Clobetasol Propionate prescription drugs?

Notes:

30. Where can I get more info about that?

Notes:

31. Does the Clobetasol Propionate medicine need to be stored in the fridge?

Notes:

32. Will my Clobetasol Propionate prescription drug have a drivers warning on it?

Notes:

33. What can I expect about the absorption of active ingredients in my Clobetasol Propionate prescription medications?

Notes:

34. Is there any form of exercise or medication you can recommend to enhance the effects of Clobetasol Propionate?

Notes:

35. Is there a better way to easily adhere to Clobetasol Propionate prescription medication regimens?

Notes:

36. What should I do if my symptoms are not relieved while taking Clobetasol Propionate medication?

Notes:

37. Where would you send your partner or children?

Notes:

38. Does switching Clobetasol Propionate prescription drugs to over the counter as I age have any negative side effects?

Notes:

39. What if I take pain medication for _____?

Notes:

40. Are there health insurers who reimburse for Clobetasol Propionate prescription drugs based on how well they work?

Notes:

41. How do I avoid getting in a place where I need so many prescription drugs to function?

Notes:

42. Is there an effective herbal alternative or supplement to Clobetasol Propionate medication?

Notes:

43. Is it safe getting pregnant while on Clobetasol Propionate medications?

Notes:

44. Can enzymes be taken when a person is on Clobetasol Propionate prescription medications?

Notes:

45. Where are others buying their Clobetasol Propionate prescription medications?

Notes:

46. Will my gender or ethnic group be denied Clobetasol Propionate medications that work better for other groups but not for my ethnic or gender group?

Notes:

47. Do enzymes interfere with Clobetasol Propionate prescription drugs?

Notes:

48. Is _____ a side effect of Clobetasol Propionate medication and is it permanent?

Notes:

49. Is it normal to feel this way?

Notes:

50. Can I safely use natural remedies and Clobetasol Propionate prescription drugs together?

Notes:

51. Do I need to prepare for the test (for example - by fasting beforehand)?

Notes:

52. Where should I get my Clobetasol Propionate prescription drugs?

Notes:

53. Where would I store my Clobetasol Propionate medications?

Notes:

54. Can assisted living patients receive 90-day supplies of medications?

Notes:

55. Will you try and keep my Clobetasol Propionate medications at a level where I can function?

Notes:

56. What are the effects of Clobetasol Propionate medications on cognition?

Notes:

57. Are extended-release (ER) opioid medications optimum pain medications?

Notes:

58. Are my Clobetasol Propionate prescription drugs FDA-approved?

Notes:

59. If I want to talk to a specialist in Clobetasol

Propionate prescription drugs, where do I go?

Notes:

CHAPTER #4: WHEN:

INTENT: When should I take or stop
taking Clobetasol Propionate and how
(When should I take it, stop taking it
and how.)

1. Could natural products be just as effective as
Clobetasol Propionate prescription medications?

Notes:

2. Can alternative medicine counter Clobetasol
Propionate prescription medication and over-the-
counters with their limited effectiveness and potential
side effects?

Notes:

3. What are the active ingredients in Clobetasol
Propionate prescription medication?

Notes:

4. Where does my Clobetasol Propionate prescription medication come from?

Notes:

5. Is there an effective way to prevent and treat without Clobetasol Propionate prescription drugs?

Notes:

6. What does one do when the only real help, the only Clobetasol Propionate medication available, no longer works?

Notes:

7. Which Clobetasol Propionate prescription drugs can be addictive?

Notes:

8. When should I stop using Clobetasol Propionate medication because of....?

Notes:

9. Could a lot of the symptoms and brain fog I get be from the Clobetasol Propionate medications themselves?

Notes:

10. When should I be on Clobetasol Propionate medication?

Notes:

11. **What medications do I need to stop and when?**

Notes:

12. **What is the difference between a natural herbal supplement and a prescription drug?**

Notes:

13. When does this Clobetasol Propionate medication expire?

Notes:

14. Is it either / or when it comes to natural medicines and Clobetasol Propionate prescription drugs?

Notes:

15. Can the nurse see me?

Notes:

16. I am paid to _____ for a living, will my performance improve or decrease while using Clobetasol Propionate prescription drugs?

Notes:

17. Do you earn bonuses based on performance?

Notes:

18. What are some great ways to help remind me when to take Clobetasol Propionate medications?

Notes:

19. How and when should I take my Clobetasol Propionate medication?

Notes:

20. When I have been on the same amount of Clobetasol Propionate medication for years – when should that be re-evaluated?

Notes:

21. Should I lock up my Clobetasol Propionate prescription drugs?

Notes:

22. If you have a Clobetasol Propionate prescription drug in your pocket, outside of the container when arrested is that considered DUI?

Notes:

23. Will I feel doped from Clobetasol Propionate?

Notes:

24. Should I expect a dependance on a medication which provides relief?

Notes:

25. Can I still take my current medications?

Notes:

26. What are the differences between generic and brand medications?

Notes:

27. When should I take this Clobetasol Propionate medicine?

Notes:

28. How does herb _____ compare to, or has an effect on, Clobetasol Propionate prescription drugs?

Notes:

29. Should I bring a list of medications and allergies?

Notes:

30. When does Clobetasol Propionate medication begin working?

Notes:

31. Is self-administration of Clobetasol Propionate medication allowed?

Notes:

32. How do you handle potential prescription drug addiction and flow-on depression?

Notes:

33. Can Clobetasol Propionate be mixed with other medications, dietary supplements, or alcohol?

Notes:

34. Do pill boxes help prevent Clobetasol Propionate

medication errors?

Notes:

35. When will I know that I am taking excessive pain medication?

Notes:

36. Are there any supplements or Clobetasol Propionate medications?

Notes:

37. When is it appropriate and safe to prescribe Clobetasol Propionate medication for my condition?

Notes:

38. How do I deal with any Clobetasol Propionate prescription medication when a side effect may be stated as 'may cause nausea or vomiting'?

Notes:

39. Can Reiki be used when taking Clobetasol

Propionate medications?

Notes:

40. Are there any known Clobetasol Propionate prescription medication and chia seeds side effects when they are combined?

Notes:

41. When might herbal and nutritional therapies be a good alternative to over-the-counter and Clobetasol Propionate prescription medications for people with my condition?

Notes:

42. Can people be guilty of DUI if they are driving under the influence of Clobetasol Propionate prescription medications?

Notes:

43. Which of my medications cause the most weight gain?

Notes:

44. When and how will I get the results?

Notes:

45. Are there any other precautions or warnings for this Clobetasol Propionate medication?

Notes:

46. When should I stop taking Clobetasol Propionate medication?

Notes:

47. When can seniors join a Clobetasol Propionate prescription drug plan?

Notes:

48. When could Clobetasol Propionate medication not be working anymore?

Notes:

49. Are these Clobetasol Propionate medications really helping?

Notes:

50. Will any of the current Clobetasol Propionate medications I am taking increase my risk for _____?

Notes:

51. Can my child have his or her Clobetasol Propionate medication administered during the school day?

Notes:

52. When did you graduate from medical school?

Notes:

53. Are generics available for all Clobetasol Propionate prescription drugs?

Notes:

54. How does a Clobetasol Propionate medication

reminder service work?

Notes:

55. How/when do I get test results?

Notes:

56. Which Clobetasol Propionate-related prescription drugs are most dangerous?

Notes:

57. Do vitamins interact with Clobetasol Propionate medications?

Notes:

58. Will Clobetasol Propionate interact with any other medicines I take - including any vitamins - herbal medicine or other complementary medicine?

Notes:

CHAPTER #5: WHY:

INTENT: Why do I need Clobetasol Propionate (Are there Alternatives. Why do I need it. Which symptoms does it medicate.)

1. Why does my family's medical history matter, and what should I do about it?

Notes:

2. Can Clobetasol Propionate medications or my health problems keep me awake?

Notes:

3. Does Clobetasol Propionate medication work?

Notes:

4. Why does a prescription drug require authorization by a qualified professional and others do not?

Notes:

5. If I take a Clobetasol Propionate medication, will it require more medication to counter the side effects?

Notes:

6. Will you keep my current medications the same?

Notes:

7. Have you heard any stories about buying Clobetasol Propionate prescription drugs over the internet?

Notes:

8. Will grapefruit affect my Clobetasol Propionate medications?

Notes:

9. Is there financial help for Clobetasol Propionate prescription drugs?

Notes:

10. Are Clobetasol Propionate prescription drugs covered?

Notes:

11. Is there a Clobetasol Propionate prescription drug guide on the internet?

Notes:

12. Why would I, while regularly taking prescription medications, have to approach grapefruit consumption with caution?

Notes:

13. Why are Clobetasol Propionate medications so popular?

Notes:

14. Is the Clobetasol Propionate medication safe?

Notes:

15. Why go the Clobetasol Propionate medication route?

Notes:

16. Why can't I buy some prescription drugs online?

Notes:

17. Why is this Clobetasol Propionate medication prescribed?

Notes:

18. Are Clobetasol Propionate medications effective?

Notes:

19. Do you know of any natural medication to

help?

Notes:

20. Why do I need Clobetasol Propionate medicine?

Notes:

21. Is Clobetasol Propionate the right medication?

Notes:

22. Will Clobetasol Propionate have an effect on nausea?

Notes:

23. Why is buying Clobetasol Propionate prescription drugs without a prescription dangerous?

Notes:

24. Why do I need to manage Clobetasol Propionate medications?

Notes:

25. Do we have to do this test now?

Notes:

26. Can you help me save money on my Clobetasol Propionate prescription medication?

Notes:

27. Could any of the Clobetasol Propionate medications contribute to impotence?

Notes:

28. Is Clobetasol Propionate medication a substitute for therapy?

Notes:

29. Why and when use acupuncture for treating pain instead of, or combined with, taking pain medication?

Notes:

30. Do I HAVE to be on Clobetasol Propionate medication?

Notes:

31. Is Clobetasol Propionate safe if taking medications for high blood pressure?

Notes:

32. Is _____ normal to get after only been taking the Clobetasol Propionate medication for a few days?

Notes:

33. Why is it important to take my Clobetasol Propionate prescription medication exactly as prescribed?

Notes:

34. Is this normal or should I see a shrink for Clobetasol Propionate medication?

Notes:

35. Is it necessary to refill my Clobetasol Propionate medication repeatedly annually?

Notes:

36. What would happen if I were suddenly unable to get access to my Clobetasol Propionate prescription drugs?

Notes:

37. Can I take Clobetasol Propionate with my other medications?

Notes:

38. Why are we doing these tests?

Notes:

39. Why is Clobetasol Propionate a prescription drug?

Notes:

40. What if my religion condones the use of Clobetasol Propionate medications?

Notes:

41. Where are Clobetasol Propionate prescription drug users getting their prescription filled locally?

Notes:

42. Can I continue to take Clobetasol Propionate prescription drugs over 10, 20 and 30 years or more?

Notes:

43. Why is Clobetasol Propionate medication prescribed?

Notes:

44. Do I have to be on more medications because of the side effects of Clobetasol Propionate?

Notes:

45. Why are you doing this test?

Notes:

46. Are all drug-drug interactions limited to Clobetasol Propionate prescription medications?

Notes:

47. Do you know all of the risks Clobetasol Propionate prescription drugs might pose?

Notes:

48. Have you instructed patients to discontinue taking their Clobetasol Propionate, or other prescription drugs?

Notes:

49. Will taking Clobetasol Propionate make me irritable?

Notes:

50. Can I take ayurvedic products with Clobetasol Propionate prescription medications?

Notes:

51. Do I need medication or surgery?

Notes:

52. Is my weight okay?

Notes:

53. Why have my bowel habits/appetite/mood/sex drive/etc changed?

Notes:

54. Why are you giving me a blood test - and what will the results tell us?

Notes:

55. Is it possible to lower my blood pressure without taking prescription drugs?

Notes:

56. Why would I need Clobetasol Propionate prescription medication reminders?

Notes:

57. Please explain, what are the differences between generic and brand Clobetasol Propionate medications?

Notes:

58. Is it probable to uncover how to deal with _____ without taking prescription medication?

Notes:

59. When is it time to think about why I'm on these Clobetasol Propionate drugs?

Notes:

CHAPTER #6: HOW:

INTENT: How will Clobetasol Propionate affect me (How will it affect me negatively. How do I know if its a problem for me.)

1. How does a person with dementia, living alone, manage her Clobetasol Propionate medication?

Notes:

2. How does Clobetasol Propionate prescription drug abuse start?

Notes:

3. How can Clobetasol Propionate medication be detected?

Notes:

4. How will I feel when I'm on Clobetasol Propionate medications?

Notes:

5. How should I use this Clobetasol Propionate medication?

Notes:

6. How should I dispose of Clobetasol Propionate prescription drugs?

Notes:

7. So how do I save money on my Clobetasol Propionate prescription drugs?

Notes:

8. How can I opt for the generic alternative Clobetasol Propionate medication that gives me the exact same results?

Notes:

9. How do I manage my Clobetasol Propionate medications?

Notes:

10. How are Clobetasol Propionate prescription drugs abused?

Notes:

11. How can I reduce or stop some of my medications?

Notes:

12. How long does a Clobetasol Propionate medication remain active in your body?

Notes:

13. How do I get better without Clobetasol Propionate medication?

Notes:

14. Are there support groups for people with this problem and how would I contact them?

Notes:

15. How about a new Clobetasol Propionate-like prescription drug?

Notes:

16. How do we order or pick up Clobetasol Propionate medications?

Notes:

17. How effective is this treatment?

Notes:

18. How will I get the test results?

Notes:

19. How do you handle children on Clobetasol

Propionate medication?

Notes:

20. How can I reduce my Clobetasol Propionate prescription drug costs?

Notes:

21. How do I read the label on my Clobetasol Propionate prescription drug package?

Notes:

22. How does Clobetasol Propionate interact with other medications?

Notes:

23. How do I dispose of Clobetasol Propionate prescription medications?

Notes:

24. How will I know if my current Clobetasol Propionate Prescription Drug coverage is as good as

the new Medicare Clobetasol Propionate Prescription Drug coverage?

Notes:

25. How common is Clobetasol Propionate prescription drug abuse?

Notes:

26. How to go about it if I want to use a lower dosage of Clobetasol Propionate?

Notes:

27. How long should I take Clobetasol Propionate medication?

Notes:

28. How will I hear about my test results?

Notes:

29. How long does the prescription drug Clobetasol Propionate stay in your system?

Notes:

30. How can I learn more about my symptoms or condition?

Notes:

31. How often will I take the Clobetasol Propionate medication?

Notes:

32. How soon should I come back?

Notes:

33. How long will it take to get the results?

Notes:

34. How many patients with my condition have you treated?

Notes:

35. How can I find a few methods that can help my condition without the use of Clobetasol Propionate prescription medication?

Notes:

36. How will Clobetasol Propionate affect the other medications that I'm taking?

Notes:

37. So I got a condition and a Clobetasol Propionate medication – how am I, as a patient, supposed to manage treatment?

Notes:

38. How to store Clobetasol Propionate medication?

Notes:

39. How is the Clobetasol Propionate medication delivered?

Notes:

40. How should I take my Clobetasol Propionate medication?

Notes:

41. How often do I need to have the test done?

Notes:

42. Do you know how long it will take me to get my Clobetasol Propionate medication?

Notes:

43. Is it probable to find out how to deal with my condition without taking Clobetasol Propionate prescription drugs?

Notes:

44. How is Clobetasol Propionate medication supposed to help me?

Notes:

45. How do I know if I have permanent hair loss due to medication?

Notes:

46. How should this Clobetasol Propionate medication be taken?

Notes:

47. How should this Clobetasol Propionate medication be stored?

Notes:

48. How long will I need the treatment for?

Notes:

49. My Clobetasol Propionate medications, just how safe are they?

Notes:

50. How do different Clobetasol Propionate-class

prescription medications work differently?

Notes:

51. How long do I need to take the Clobetasol Propionate medicine for?

Notes:

52. Are there drugs to lift my mood, and how can this be achieved without prescription medications?

Notes:

53. How can Clobetasol Propionate prescription drug abuse be recognized and stopped?

Notes:

54. How do I take this Clobetasol Propionate medication?

Notes:

55. How often is the Clobetasol Propionate

medication taken?

Notes:

56. How accurate are the results of the test?

Notes:

57. How quickly do I have to start the treatment?

Notes:

58. How wide-ranging is the Clobetasol Propionate prescription drug coverage?

Notes:

59. How many surgeries do you perform each year?

Notes:

60. How's my weight?

Notes:

61. How long do I have to take Clobetasol Propionate medication?

Notes:

62. How is the test done?

Notes:

63. How will I know if the Clobetasol Propionate prescription and over-the-counter medications I take are interacting properly?

Notes:

64. State prescription drug price web sites, how useful are they to me as a Clobetasol Propionate consumer?

Notes:

65. How should I take this Clobetasol Propionate medication?

Notes:

66. How do I manage multiple prescription medications together with Clobetasol Propionate?

Notes:

67. How can I support my bone health naturally with and without medication?

Notes:

68. How long will the effect of Clobetasol Propionate medication last?

Notes:

69. How will Clobetasol Propionate affect my sleeping pattern?

Notes:

70. So how do you know if you, or someone you love is having problems with Clobetasol Propionate prescription drug abuse?

Notes:

71. How long is it likely to last?

Notes:

72. How can I dispose of my Clobetasol Propionate prescription drugs safely?

Notes:

73. How do generic medications compare in quality to brand name drugs?

Notes:

74. In case I need pain relief, how can I get access to medical cannabis?

Notes:

75. How soon do I need to have the test?

Notes:

76. How can I make sure I am sufficiently stocked with the Clobetasol Propionate prescription medications I

need?

Notes:

77. How can my mental state successfully improve using medication or therapy?

Notes:

78. How do the police suspect impairment by Clobetasol Propionate prescription medication?

Notes:

79. How serious is this condition?

Notes:

80. How long does the Clobetasol Propionate medication last?

Notes:

CHAPTER #7: HOW MUCH:

INTENT: How much will taking Clobetasol Propionate cost me (In money and Clobetasol Propionate's effect on quality of life.)

1. Can you explain my options for Medicare, Medicare/Medicaid, Disability, Supplemental Insurance, Part D Prescription Drug Plans, or Medicare Billings?

Notes:

2. How much will the plan cover for Clobetasol Propionate prescription drugs?

Notes:

3. Should I join a Medicare Prescription Drug Plan even if I don't take many prescription drugs?

Notes:

4. How much will the test cost?

Notes:

5. Where can one undertake Clobetasol Propionate prescription drug addiction treatment?

Notes:

6. Is it covered by Medicare - my concession or Veterans Affairs card or my private health insurance?

Notes:

7. Should I be concerned about all the Clobetasol Propionate medication I need to take to stay on top of my health problems?

Notes:

8. How much do I need to really understand about the interactions of my Clobetasol Propionate prescription

drugs?

Notes:

9. May I bring multiple prescription medications to take while I am in custody?

Notes:

10. Will I require any Clobetasol Propionate prescription drugs?

Notes:

11. Will Medicare be enough to cover the cost of my medical care, especially Clobetasol Propionate prescription drugs?

Notes:

12. Do some Clobetasol Propionate prescription drugs cost more or have additional requirements for coverage?

Notes:

13. Which part of Medicare will cover my Clobetasol Propionate prescription drugs?

Notes:

14. Are there any side effects of taking Clobetasol Propionate?

Notes:

15. Are Clobetasol Propionate medications toxic?

Notes:

16. Do we have to do this now - or can we revisit it later?

Notes:

17. How much Clobetasol Propionate prescription medication can I order from my pharmacy at one time?

Notes:

18. Are my prescription drugs also available in a

generic version?

Notes:

19. Can or should I take my Clobetasol Propionate medications at breakfast with my grapefruit juice?

Notes:

20. How much will my Clobetasol Propionate prescription drugs cost me?

Notes:

21. When you prescribe Clobetasol Propionate prescription medication for my condition, how do you weigh the side effects?

Notes:

22. How much is Medicare Clobetasol Propionate prescription drug coverage worth?

Notes:

23. How much am I likely to spend on Clobetasol

Propionate prescription drugs?

Notes:

24. I am on prescription Clobetasol Propionate medication, can I still detox?

Notes:

25. If I have been taking the same prescription drugs for a long time, when is it time to evaluate?

Notes:

26. Regarding dosage, exactly how much of Clobetasol Propionate can I take?

Notes:

27. What are the Clobetasol Propionate prescription drug prices?

Notes:

28. How much should I be charged for my Clobetasol Propionate prescription medications?

Notes:

29. How do Clobetasol Propionate prescription drugs work?

Notes:

30. Did you wash your hands?

Notes:

31. How much does it normally cost to get the surgery done, including all Clobetasol Propionate medications and tests (ultrasounds,x-rays,medicines, hospital stay)?

Notes:

32. Am I am worrying too much?

Notes:

33. How much experience with this test or procedure do you have?

Notes:

34. How much will it cost, will the cost be covered by the PBS - my concession or Veterans Affairs card or by private health insurance?

Notes:

35. How much will this cost me?

Notes:

36. How much does Clobetasol Propionate cost?

Notes:

37. Are there any contraindications with Clobetasol Propionate to other medications?

Notes:

38. Is Clobetasol Propionate a medication?

Notes:

39. Do Clobetasol Propionate prescription drugs create new mental problems?

Notes:

40. Is Clobetasol Propionate compatible with my current prescribed medication?

Notes:

41. How much can I use this Clobetasol Propionate prescription drug plan?

Notes:

42. Just how much do you know about the numerous types of Clobetasol Propionate medications for the different types of my condition?

Notes:

43. How do I get the Medicare Clobetasol Propionate prescription drug benefit?

Notes:

44. How much do the Clobetasol Propionate prescription drugs cost in this plan as compared to other plans?

Notes:

45. Can you take expired Clobetasol Propionate medications or not?

Notes:

46. How do I know how much my Clobetasol Propionate prescription medication will be?

Notes:

47. If I get concerned with the high cost of medical care and Clobetasol Propionate prescriptions drugs, will you help me explore my options for a more natural approach like seeking help from acupuncturists, naturopaths, chiropractors?

Notes:

48. Is there a generic version of the Clobetasol Propionate medication?

Notes:

49. Will the cost be covered by Medicare - my concession or Veterans Affairs card or by private health insurance?

Notes:

50. Can I take _____ with Clobetasol Propionate prescription drugs?

Notes:

51. How much Clobetasol Propionate medication can be brought through customs in case I travel?

Notes:

52. Is there a Medicare Advantage plan provider who will cover my Clobetasol Propionate prescription drug costs during the donut hole?

Notes:

53. How much will the treatment cost?

Notes:

54. I Googled my symptoms and read this. Is it accurate?

Notes:

55. Are the brands of Clobetasol Propionate prescription drugs I take covered?

Notes:

56. If I need a surgery and I did go ahead with the surgery, how might that affect the Clobetasol Propionate medications I take?

Notes:

57. Do you think that I may have or get a problem with Clobetasol Propionate medications?

Notes:

58. How to get my Clobetasol Propionate medication increased?

Notes:

59. What if I start depending on antidepressants, alcohol, or other medications to calm me down or help me sleep?

Notes:

Index

Made in the USA
Columbia, SC
21 October 2020